SUPER VEGAN CUISINE 2022

RECIPES TO CLEANSE YOUR BODY AND MIND

HENRY SPEED

Table of Contents

3

4

Artichoke Capers and Artichoke Heart Salad

Ingredients:

1 artichoke, rinsed, patted and shredded

½ cup capers

½ cup artichoke hearts

Dressing

2 tbsp. white wine vinegar

4 tablespoons extra virgin olive oil

Freshly ground black pepper

3/4 cup finely ground almonds

Sea salt

Prep

Combine all of the dressing ingredients in a food processor.

Toss with the rest of the ingredients and combine well.

Mixed Greens Baby Corn and Artichoke Heart Salad

Ingredients:

1 bunch Mesclun, rinsed, patted and shredded

½ cup canned baby corn

½ cup artichoke hearts

Dressing

2 tbsp. white wine vinegar

4 tablespoons extra virgin olive oil

Freshly ground black pepper

3/4 cup finely ground peanuts

Sea salt

Prep

Combine all of the dressing ingredients in a food processor.

Toss with the rest of the ingredients and combine well.

Romaine Lettuce with Tomatillo Dressing

Ingredients:

1 head Romaine lettuce, shredded

4 large tomatoes, seeded and chopped

4 radishes, thinly sliced

Dressing

6 tomatillos, rinsed and halved

1 jalapeno, halved

1 white onion, quartered

2 tablespoons extra virgin olive oil

Kosher salt and freshly ground black pepper

1/2 teaspoon ground cumin

1 cup Dairy free cream cheese

2 tablespoons fresh lemon juice

Prep/Cook

Preheat the oven to 400 degrees F.

For the dressing, place the tomatillos, jalapeno and onion on a cookie sheet.

Drizzle with olive oil and sprinkle with salt and pepper.

Roast in the oven for 25- 30 min. until vegetables begin to brown and slightly darken.

Transfer to a food processor and let it cool then blend.

Add the rest of the ingredients and refrigerate for an hour.

Toss with the rest of the ingredients and combine well.

Greek Romaine Lettuce and Tomato Salad

Ingredients:

1 head romaine lettuce, chopped

4 whole ripe tomatoes, cut into 6 wedges each, then each wedge cut in half

1 whole medium cucumber, peeled, cut into fourths lengthwise, and diced into large chunks

1/2 whole white onion, sliced very thin

30 whole pitted green olives, cut in half lengthwise, plus 6 olives, chopped fine

6 ounces crumbled vegan cheese

Fresh parsley leaves, roughly chopped

Dressing

1/4 cup extra virgin olive oil

2 tablespoons white wine vinegar

1 teaspoon sugar, or more to taste

1 clove garlic, minced

Salt and freshly ground black pepper

Juice of ½ lemon

Sea salt

Prep

Combine all of the dressing ingredients in a food processor and blend.

Season with more salt if necessary.

Toss all of the ingredients together.

Plum Tomato and Cucumber Salad

Ingredients:

5 medium plum tomatoes, halved lengthwise, seeded, and thinly sliced
1/4 white onion, peeled, halved lengthwise, and thinly sliced
1 large cucumber, halved lengthwise and thinly sliced

Dressing
¼ cup extra-virgin olive oil
2 splashes white wine vinegar
Coarse salt and black pepper

Prep
Combine all of the dressing ingredients.

Toss with the rest of the ingredients and combine well.

Enoki Mushroom and Cucumber Salad

Ingredients:

15 Enoki Mushrooms, thinly sliced

1/4 white onion, peeled, halved lengthwise, and thinly sliced

1 large cucumber, halved lengthwise and thinly sliced

Dressing

¼ cup extra-virgin olive oil

2 splashes white wine vinegar

Coarse salt and black pepper

Prep

Combine all of the dressing ingredients.

Toss with the rest of the ingredients and combine well.

Tomato and Zucchini Salad

Ingredients:

5 medium tomatoes, halved lengthwise, seeded, and thinly sliced

1/4 white onion, peeled, halved lengthwise, and thinly sliced

1 large Zucchini halved lengthwise ,thinly sliced & blanched

Dressing

¼ cup extra-virgin olive oil

2 tbsp. apple cider vinegar

Coarse salt and black pepper

Prep

Combine all of the dressing ingredients.

Toss with the rest of the ingredients and combine well.

Tomatillos with Cucumber Salad

Ingredients:

10 Tomatillos, halved lengthwise, seeded, and thinly sliced

1/4 white onion, peeled, halved lengthwise, and thinly sliced

1 large cucumber, halved lengthwise and thinly sliced

Dressing

¼ cup extra-virgin olive oil

2 splashes white wine vinegar

Coarse salt and black pepper

Prep

Combine all of the dressing ingredients.

Toss with the rest of the ingredients and combine well.

Plum Tomato and Onion Salad

Ingredients:

5 medium plum tomatoes, halved lengthwise, seeded, and thinly sliced

1/4 white onion, peeled, halved lengthwise, and thinly sliced

1 large cucumber, halved lengthwise and thinly sliced

Dressing

¼ cup extra-virgin olive oil

2 tbsp. apple cider vinegar

Coarse salt and black pepper

Prep

Combine all of the dressing ingredients.

Toss with the rest of the ingredients and combine well.

Zucchini and tomato Salad

Ingredients:

5 medium tomatoes, halved lengthwise, seeded, and thinly sliced

1/4 white onion, peeled, halved lengthwise, and thinly sliced

1 large Zucchini halved lengthwise ,thinly sliced and blanched

Dressing

¼ cup extra-virgin olive oil

2 splashes white wine vinegar

Coarse salt and black pepper

Prep

Combine all of the dressing ingredients.

Toss with the rest of the ingredients and combine well.

Heirloom Tomato Salad

Ingredients:

3 Heirloom tomatoes, halved lengthwise, seeded, and thinly sliced

1/4 white onion, peeled, halved lengthwise, and thinly sliced

1 large cucumber, halved lengthwise and thinly sliced

Dressing

¼ cup extra-virgin olive oil

2 splashes white wine vinegar

Coarse salt and black pepper

Prep

Combine all of the dressing ingredients.

Toss with the rest of the ingredients and combine well.

Enoki Mushroom Salad

Ingredients:

15 Enoki Mushrooms, thinly sliced

1/4 white onion, peeled, halved lengthwise, and thinly sliced

1 large cucumber, halved lengthwise and thinly sliced

Dressing

¼ cup extra-virgin olive oil

2 tbsp. apple cider vinegar

Coarse salt and black pepper

Prep

Combine all of the dressing ingredients.

Toss with the rest of the ingredients and combine well.

Artichoke Heart and Plum Tomato Salad

Ingredients:

6 Artichoke Hearts (Canned)

5 medium plum tomatoes, halved lengthwise, seeded, and thinly sliced

1/4 white onion, peeled, halved lengthwise, and thinly sliced

1 large cucumber, halved lengthwise and thinly sliced

Dressing

¼ cup extra-virgin olive oil

2 splashes white wine vinegar

Coarse salt and black pepper

Prep

Combine all of the dressing ingredients.

Toss with the rest of the ingredients and combine well.

Baby Corn and Plum Tomato Salad

Ingredients:

½ cup canned baby corn

5 medium plum tomatoes, halved lengthwise, seeded, and thinly sliced

1/4 white onion, peeled, halved lengthwise, and thinly sliced

1 large Zucchini halved lengthwise ,thinly sliced and blanched

Dressing

¼ cup extra-virgin olive oil

2 splashes white wine vinegar

Coarse salt and black pepper

Prep

Combine all of the dressing ingredients.

Toss with the rest of the ingredients and combine well.

Mixed Greens and Tomato Salad

Ingredients:

1 bunch Meslcun, rinsed and drained

5 medium tomatoes, halved lengthwise, seeded, and thinly sliced

1/4 white onion, peeled, halved lengthwise, and thinly sliced

1 large cucumber, halved lengthwise and thinly sliced

Dressing

¼ cup extra-virgin olive oil

2 tbsp. apple cider vinegar

Coarse salt and black pepper

Prep

Combine all of the dressing ingredients.

Toss with the rest of the ingredients and combine well.

Romaine Lettuce and Plum Tomato Salad

Ingredients:

1 bunch Romaine Lettuce, rinsed and drained

5 medium plum tomatoes, halved lengthwise, seeded, and thinly sliced

1/4 white onion, peeled, halved lengthwise, and thinly sliced

1 large cucumber, halved lengthwise and thinly sliced

Dressing

¼ cup extra-virgin olive oil

2 splashes white wine vinegar

Coarse salt and black pepper

Prep

Combine all of the dressing ingredients.

Toss with the rest of the ingredients and combine well.

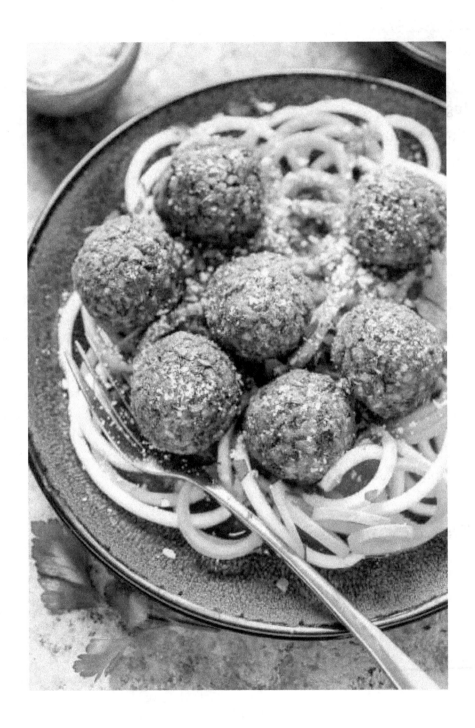

Endive and Enoki Mushroom Salad

Ingredients:

1 bunch Endive, rinsed and drained

15 Enoki Mushrooms, thinly sliced

1/4 white onion, peeled, halved lengthwise, and thinly sliced

1 large cucumber, halved lengthwise and thinly sliced

Dressing

¼ cup extra-virgin olive oil

2 splashes white wine vinegar

Coarse salt and black pepper

Prep

Combine all of the dressing ingredients.

Toss with the rest of the ingredients and combine well.

Artichoke and Tomato Salad

Ingredients:

1 Artichoke, rinsed and drained

5 medium tomatoes, halved lengthwise, seeded, and thinly sliced

1/4 white onion, peeled, halved lengthwise, and thinly sliced

1 large Zucchini halved lengthwise ,thinly sliced and blanched

Dressing

¼ cup extra-virgin olive oil

2 splashes white wine vinegar

Coarse salt and black pepper

Prep

Combine all of the dressing ingredients.

Toss with the rest of the ingredients and combine well.

Kale and Heirloom Tomato Salad

Ingredients:

1 bunch Kale, rinsed and drained

3 Heirloom tomatoes, halved lengthwise, seeded, and thinly sliced

1/4 white onion, peeled, halved lengthwise, and thinly sliced

1 large cucumber, halved lengthwise and thinly sliced

Dressing

¼ cup extra-virgin olive oil

2 tbsp. apple cider vinegar

Coarse salt and black pepper

Prep

Combine all of the dressing ingredients.

Toss with the rest of the ingredients and combine well.

Spinach and Tomatillo Salad

Ingredients:

1 bunch Spinach, rinsed and drained

10 Tomatillos, halved lengthwise, seeded, and thinly sliced

1/4 white onion, peeled, halved lengthwise, and thinly sliced

1 large cucumber, halved lengthwise and thinly sliced

Dressing

¼ cup extra-virgin olive oil

2 splashes white wine vinegar

Coarse salt and black pepper

Prep

Combine all of the dressing ingredients.

Toss with the rest of the ingredients and combine well.

Mesclun and Enoki Mushroom Salad

Ingredients:

1 bunch Meslcun, rinsed and drained

15 Enoki Mushrooms, thinly sliced

1/4 white onion, peeled, halved lengthwise, and thinly sliced

1 large cucumber, halved lengthwise and thinly sliced

Dressing

¼ cup extra-virgin olive oil

2 splashes white wine vinegar

Coarse salt and black pepper

Prep

Combine all of the dressing ingredients.

Toss with the rest of the ingredients and combine well.

Romaine Lettuce and Cucumber Salad

Ingredients:

1 bunch Romaine Lettuce, rinsed and drained

5 medium plum tomatoes, halved lengthwise, seeded, and thinly sliced

1/4 white onion, peeled, halved lengthwise, and thinly sliced

1 large cucumber, halved lengthwise and thinly sliced

Dressing

¼ cup extra-virgin olive oil

2 tbsp. apple cider vinegar

Coarse salt and black pepper

Prep

Combine all of the dressing ingredients.

Toss with the rest of the ingredients and combine well.

Kale Spinach and Zucchini Salad

Ingredients:

1 bunch Kale, rinsed and drained

1 bunch Spinach, rinsed and drained

1/4 white onion, peeled, halved lengthwise, and thinly sliced

1 large Zucchini halved lengthwise ,thinly sliced and blanched

Dressing

¼ cup extra-virgin olive oil

2 splashes white wine vinegar

Coarse salt and black pepper

Prep

Combine all of the dressing ingredients.

Toss with the rest of the ingredients and combine well.

Artichoke Kale and Enoki Mushroom Salad

Ingredients:

1 Artichoke, rinsed and drained

1 bunch Kale, rinsed and drained

15 Enoki Mushrooms, thinly sliced

1/4 white onion, peeled, halved lengthwise, and thinly sliced

1 large cucumber, halved lengthwise and thinly sliced

Dressing

¼ cup extra-virgin olive oil

2 splashes white wine vinegar

Coarse salt and black pepper

Prep

Combine all of the dressing ingredients.

Toss with the rest of the ingredients and combine well.

Endive and Artichoke Salad

Ingredients:

1 bunch Endive, rinsed and drained

1 Artichoke, rinsed and drained

1 large cucumber, halved lengthwise and thinly sliced

Dressing

¼ cup extra-virgin olive oil

2 splashes white wine vinegar

Coarse salt and black pepper

Prep

Combine all of the dressing ingredients.

Toss with the rest of the ingredients and combine well.

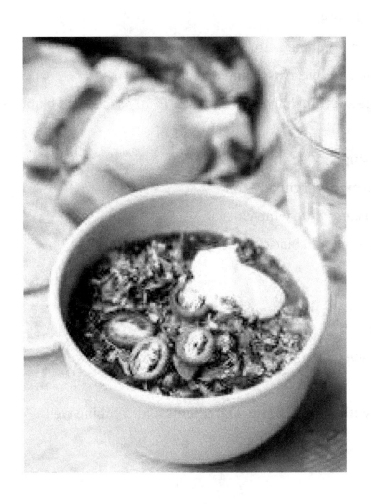

Endive and Zucchini Salad

Ingredients:

1 bunch Romaine Lettuce, rinsed and drained

1 bunch Endive, rinsed and drained

1 large Zucchini halved lengthwise, thinly sliced and blanched

Dressing

¼ cup extra-virgin olive oil

2 splashes white wine vinegar

Coarse salt and black pepper

Prep

Combine all of the dressing ingredients.

Toss with the rest of the ingredients and combine well.

Mesclun and Romaine Lettuce Salad

Ingredients:

1 bunch Meslcun, rinsed and drained

1 bunch Romaine Lettuce, rinsed and drained

1/4 white onion, peeled, halved lengthwise, and thinly sliced

1 large cucumber, halved lengthwise and thinly sliced

Dressing

¼ cup extra-virgin olive oil

2 tbsp. apple cider vinegar

Coarse salt and black pepper

Prep

Combine all of the dressing ingredients.

Toss with the rest of the ingredients and combine well.

Mixed Green and Tomatillo Salad

Ingredients:

1 bunch Meslcun, rinsed and drained

1 bunch Romaine Lettuce, rinsed and drained

10 Tomatillos, halved lengthwise, seeded, and thinly sliced

1/4 white onion, peeled, halved lengthwise, and thinly sliced

1 large Zucchini halved lengthwise ,thinly sliced and blanched

Dressing

¼ cup extra-virgin olive oil

2 splashes white wine vinegar

Coarse salt and black pepper

Prep

Combine all of the dressing ingredients.

Toss with the rest of the ingredients and combine well.

Romaine Lettuce and Endive Salad

Ingredients:

1 bunch Romaine Lettuce, rinsed and drained

1 bunch Endive, rinsed and drained

5 medium plum tomatoes, halved lengthwise, seeded, and thinly sliced

1/4 white onion, peeled, halved lengthwise, and thinly sliced

1 large cucumber, halved lengthwise and thinly sliced

Dressing

¼ cup extra-virgin olive oil

2 splashes white wine vinegar

Coarse salt and black pepper

Prep

Combine all of the dressing ingredients.

Toss with the rest of the ingredients and combine well.

Artichoke and Kale Salad

Ingredients:

1 Artichoke, rinsed and drained

1 bunch Kale, rinsed and drained

3 Heirloom tomatoes, halved lengthwise, seeded, and thinly sliced

1/4 white onion, peeled, halved lengthwise, and thinly sliced

1 large cucumber, halved lengthwise and thinly sliced

Dressing

¼ cup extra-virgin olive oil

2 splashes white wine vinegar

Coarse salt and black pepper

Prep

Combine all of the dressing ingredients.

Toss with the rest of the ingredients and combine well.

Kale and Spinach Salad

Ingredients:

1 bunch Kale, rinsed and drained

1 bunch Spinach, rinsed and drained

15 Enoki Mushrooms, thinly sliced

1/4 white onion, peeled, halved lengthwise, and thinly sliced

1 large cucumber, halved lengthwise and thinly sliced

Dressing

¼ cup extra-virgin olive oil

2 splashes white wine vinegar

Coarse salt and black pepper

Prep

Combine all of the dressing ingredients.

Toss with the rest of the ingredients and combine well.

Carrots and Plum Tomato Salad

Ingredients:

1 cup baby carrots, chopped

5 medium plum tomatoes, halved lengthwise, seeded, and thinly sliced

1/4 white onion, peeled, halved lengthwise, and thinly sliced

1 large cucumber, halved lengthwise and thinly sliced

Dressing

¼ cup extra-virgin olive oil

2 tbsp. apple cider vinegar

Coarse salt and black pepper

Prep

Combine all of the dressing ingredients.

Toss with the rest of the ingredients and combine well.

Corn and Plum Tomato Salad

Ingredients:

1 cup baby corn (canned), drained

5 medium plum tomatoes, halved lengthwise, seeded, and thinly sliced

1/4 white onion, peeled, halved lengthwise, and thinly sliced

1 large Zucchini halved lengthwise ,thinly sliced and blanched

Dressing

¼ cup extra-virgin olive oil

2 splashes white wine vinegar

Coarse salt and black pepper

Prep

Combine all of the dressing ingredients.

Toss with the rest of the ingredients and combine well.

Mixed Green and Baby Carrot Salad

Ingredients:

1 bunch Meslcun, rinsed and drained

1 cup baby carrots, chopped

1 large cucumber, halved lengthwise and thinly sliced

Dressing

¼ cup extra-virgin olive oil

2 splashes white wine vinegar

Coarse salt and black pepper

Prep

Combine all of the dressing ingredients.

Toss with the rest of the ingredients and combine well.

Romaine Lettuce and Baby Corn Salad

Ingredients:

1 bunch Romaine Lettuce, rinsed and drained

1 cup baby corn (canned), drained

1 large cucumber, halved lengthwise and thinly sliced

Dressing

¼ cup extra-virgin olive oil

2 splashes white wine vinegar

Coarse salt and black pepper

Prep

Combine all of the dressing ingredients.

Toss with the rest of the ingredients and combine well.

Baby Corn and Endive Salad

Ingredients:

1 cup baby corn (canned), drained

1 bunch Endive, rinsed and drained

1/4 white onion, peeled, halved lengthwise, and thinly sliced

1 large Zucchini halved lengthwise ,thinly sliced and blanched

Dressing

¼ cup extra-virgin olive oil

2 tbsp. apple cider vinegar

Coarse salt and black pepper

Prep

Combine all of the dressing ingredients.

Toss with the rest of the ingredients and combine well.

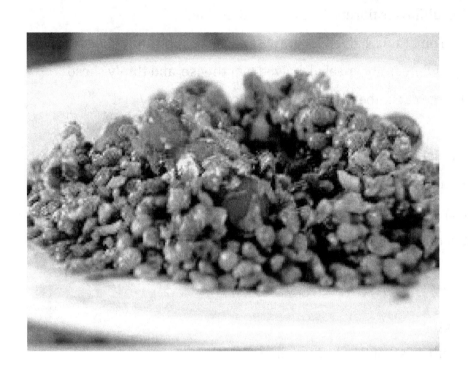

51

Cauliflower and Tomatillo Salad

Ingredients:

9 cauliflower florets, blanched and drained

10 Tomatillos, halved lengthwise, seeded, and thinly sliced

1/4 white onion, peeled, halved lengthwise, and thinly sliced

1 large cucumber, halved lengthwise and thinly sliced

Dressing

¼ cup extra-virgin olive oil

2 splashes white wine vinegar

Coarse salt and black pepper

Prep

Combine all of the dressing ingredients.

Toss with the rest of the ingredients and combine well.

Broccoli and Tomatillo Salad

Ingredients:

8 broccoli florets, blanched and drained

10 Tomatillos, halved lengthwise, seeded, and thinly sliced

1/4 white onion, peeled, halved lengthwise, and thinly sliced

1 large cucumber, halved lengthwise and thinly sliced

Dressing

¼ cup extra-virgin olive oil

2 splashes white wine vinegar

Coarse salt and black pepper

Prep

Combine all of the dressing ingredients.

Toss with the rest of the ingredients and combine well.

Spinach and Cauliflower Salad

Ingredients:

1 bunch Spinach, rinsed and drained

9 cauliflower florets, blanched and drained

1 large Zucchini halved lengthwise ,thinly sliced and blanched

Dressing

¼ cup extra-virgin olive oil

2 splashes white wine vinegar

Coarse salt and black pepper

Prep

Combine all of the dressing ingredients.

Toss with the rest of the ingredients and combine well.

Kale and Broccoli Salad

Ingredients:

1 bunch Kale, rinsed and drained

8 broccoli florets, blanched and drained

1 large cucumber, halved lengthwise and thinly sliced

Dressing

¼ cup extra-virgin olive oil

2 splashes white wine vinegar

Coarse salt and black pepper

Prep

Combine all of the dressing ingredients.

Toss with the rest of the ingredients and combine well.

Kale Spinach &Broccoli Salad

Ingredients:

1 bunch Kale, rinsed and drained

8 broccoli florets, blanched and drained

1 bunch Spinach, rinsed and drained

Dressing

¼ cup extra-virgin olive oil

2 splashes white wine vinegar

Coarse salt and black pepper

Prep

Combine all of the dressing ingredients.

Toss with the rest of the ingredients and combine well.

Artichoke Kale and Broccoli Salad

Ingredients:

1 Artichoke, rinsed and drained

1 bunch Kale, rinsed and drained

8 broccoli florets, blanched and drained

Dressing

¼ cup extra-virgin olive oil

2 splashes white wine vinegar

Coarse salt and black pepper

Prep

Combine all of the dressing ingredients.

Toss with the rest of the ingredients and combine well.

Baby Corn and Endive Salad

Ingredients:

1 cup baby corn (canned), drained

1 bunch Endive, rinsed and drained

1 Artichoke, rinsed and drained

Dressing

¼ cup extra-virgin olive oil

2 tbsp. apple cider vinegar

Coarse salt and black pepper

Prep

Combine all of the dressing ingredients.

Toss with the rest of the ingredients and combine well.

Mixed Green and Baby Carrot Salad

Ingredients:

1 bunch Meslcun, rinsed and drained

1 cup baby carrots, chopped

1 bunch Romaine Lettuce, rinsed and drained

Dressing

¼ cup extra-virgin olive oil

2 splashes white wine vinegar

Coarse salt and black pepper

Prep

Combine all of the dressing ingredients.

Toss with the rest of the ingredients and combine well.

Tomatillo and Baby Corn Salad

Ingredients:

10 Tomatillos, halved lengthwise, seeded, and thinly sliced

1 cup baby corn (canned), drained

1 bunch Endive, rinsed and drained

1 Artichoke, rinsed and drained

Dressing

¼ cup extra-virgin olive oil

2 splashes white wine vinegar

Coarse salt and black pepper

Prep

Combine all of the dressing ingredients.

Toss with the rest of the ingredients and combine well.

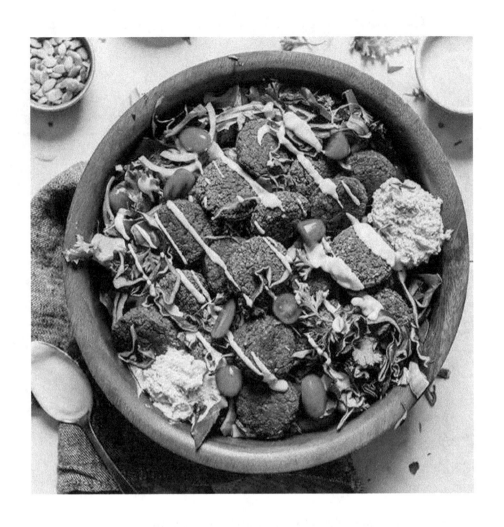

Enoki and Baby Corn Salad

Ingredients:

15 Enoki Mushrooms, thinly sliced

1 cup baby corn (canned), drained

1 bunch Endive, rinsed and drained

1 Artichoke, rinsed and drained

Dressing

¼ cup extra-virgin olive oil

2 tbsp. apple cider vinegar

Coarse salt and black pepper

Prep

Combine all of the dressing ingredients.

Toss with the rest of the ingredients and combine well.

Heirloom Tomato Endive and Artichoke Salad

Ingredients:

3 Heirloom tomatoes, halved lengthwise, seeded, and thinly sliced

1 bunch Endive, rinsed and drained

1 Artichoke, rinsed and drained

1 bunch Kale, rinsed and drained

Dressing

¼ cup extra-virgin olive oil

2 splashes white wine vinegar

Coarse salt and black pepper

Prep

Combine all of the dressing ingredients.

Toss with the rest of the ingredients and combine well.

Kale Plum Tomatoes and Onion Salad

Ingredients:

1 bunch of kale, rinsed and drained

5 medium plum tomatoes, halved lengthwise, seeded, and thinly sliced

1/4 white onion, peeled, halved lengthwise, and thinly sliced

1 large cucumber, halved lengthwise and thinly sliced

Dressing

¼ cup extra-virgin olive oil

2 splashes white wine vinegar

Coarse salt and black pepper

Prep

Combine all of the dressing ingredients.

Toss with the rest of the ingredients and combine well.

Spinach Plum Tomatoes and Onion Salad

Ingredients:

1 bunch of spinach, rinsed and drained

5 medium plum tomatoes, halved lengthwise, seeded, and thinly sliced

1/4 white onion, peeled, halved lengthwise, and thinly sliced

1 large cucumber, halved lengthwise and thinly sliced

Dressing

¼ cup extra-virgin olive oil

2 splashes white wine vinegar

Coarse salt and black pepper

Prep

Combine all of the dressing ingredients.

Toss with the rest of the ingredients and combine well.

Watercress and Zucchini Salad

Ingredients:

1 bunch of watercress, rinsed and drained

5 medium plum tomatoes, halved lengthwise, seeded, and thinly sliced

1/4 white onion, peeled, halved lengthwise, and thinly sliced

1 large Zucchini halved lengthwise ,thinly sliced and blanched

Dressing

¼ cup extra-virgin olive oil

2 tbsp. apple cider vinegar

Coarse salt and black pepper

Prep

Combine all of the dressing ingredients.

Toss with the rest of the ingredients and combine well.

Mangoes tomatoes and Cucumber Salad

Ingredients:

1 cup of cubed mangoes

5 medium plum tomatoes, halved lengthwise, seeded, and thinly sliced

1/4 white onion, peeled, halved lengthwise, and thinly sliced

1 large cucumber, halved lengthwise and thinly sliced

Dressing

¼ cup extra-virgin olive oil

2 splashes white wine vinegar

Coarse salt and black pepper

Prep

Combine all of the dressing ingredients.

Toss with the rest of the ingredients and combine well.

Peaches Tomatoes and Onion Salad

Ingredients:

1 cup of cubed peaches

5 medium tomatoes, halved lengthwise, seeded, and thinly sliced

1/4 white onion, peeled, halved lengthwise, and thinly sliced

1 large cucumber, halved lengthwise and thinly sliced

Dressing

¼ cup extra-virgin olive oil

2 splashes white wine vinegar

Coarse salt and black pepper

Prep

Combine all of the dressing ingredients.

Toss with the rest of the ingredients and combine well.

Black Grapes Tomatillo and White Onion

Ingredients:

12 pcs. black grapes

10 Tomatillos, halved lengthwise, seeded, and thinly sliced

1/4 white onion, peeled, halved lengthwise, and thinly sliced

1 large cucumber, halved lengthwise and thinly sliced

Dressing

¼ cup extra-virgin olive oil

2 splashes white wine vinegar

Coarse salt and black pepper

Prep

Combine all of the dressing ingredients.

Toss with the rest of the ingredients and combine well.

Red Grapes Tomatillo and Zucchini Salad

Ingredients:

10 pcs. red grapes

3 Heirloom tomatoes, halved lengthwise, seeded, and thinly sliced

1/4 white onion, peeled, halved lengthwise, and thinly sliced

1 large Zucchini halved lengthwise ,thinly sliced and blanched

Dressing

¼ cup extra-virgin olive oil

2 splashes white wine vinegar

Coarse salt and black pepper

Prep

Combine all of the dressing ingredients.

Toss with the rest of the ingredients and combine well.

Red Cabbage Plum Tomatoes and Onion Salad

Ingredients:

1/2 medium red cabbage, sliced thinly

5 medium plum tomatoes, halved lengthwise, seeded, and thinly sliced

1/4 white onion, peeled, halved lengthwise, and thinly sliced

1 large cucumber, halved lengthwise and thinly sliced

Dressing

¼ cup extra-virgin olive oil

2 tbsp. apple cider vinegar

Coarse salt and black pepper

Prep

Combine all of the dressing ingredients.

Toss with the rest of the ingredients and combine well.

Ingredients:

1/2 medium Napa cabbage, sliced thinly

5 medium plum tomatoes, halved lengthwise, seeded, and thinly sliced

1/4 white onion, peeled, halved lengthwise, and thinly sliced

1 large cucumber, halved lengthwise and thinly sliced

Dressing

¼ cup extra-virgin olive oil

2 tbsp. apple cider vinegar

Coarse salt and black pepper

Prep

Combine all of the dressing ingredients.

Toss with the rest of the ingredients and combine well.

Red and Napa Cabbage Salad

Ingredients:

1/2 medium red cabbage, sliced thinly

1/2 medium Napa cabbage, sliced thinly

1/4 white onion, peeled, halved lengthwise, and thinly sliced

1 large Zucchini halved lengthwise ,thinly sliced and blanched

Dressing

¼ cup extra-virgin olive oil

2 splashes white wine vinegar

Coarse salt and black pepper

Prep

Combine all of the dressing ingredients.

Toss with the rest of the ingredients and combine well.

Black and Red Grape Salad

Ingredients:

12 pcs. black grapes

10 pcs. red grapes

1/4 white onion, peeled, halved lengthwise, and thinly sliced

1 large cucumber, halved lengthwise and thinly sliced

Dressing

¼ cup extra-virgin olive oil

2 splashes white wine vinegar

Coarse salt and black pepper

Prep

Combine all of the dressing ingredients.

Toss with the rest of the ingredients and combine well.

Mangoes Peaches and Cucumber Salad

Ingredients:

1 cup of cubed mangoes

1 cup of cubed peaches

1/4 white onion, peeled, halved lengthwise, and thinly sliced

1 large cucumber, halved lengthwise and thinly sliced

Dressing

¼ cup extra-virgin olive oil

2 splashes white wine vinegar

Coarse salt and black pepper

Prep

Combine all of the dressing ingredients.

Toss with the rest of the ingredients and combine well.

Watercress Enoki Mushroom and Zucchini Salad

Ingredients:

1 bunch of watercress, rinsed and drained

15 Enoki Mushrooms, thinly sliced

1/4 white onion, peeled, halved lengthwise, and thinly sliced

1 large Zucchini halved lengthwise ,thinly sliced and blanched

Dressing

¼ cup extra-virgin olive oil

2 splashes white wine vinegar

Coarse salt and black pepper

Prep

Combine all of the dressing ingredients.

Toss with the rest of the ingredients and combine well.

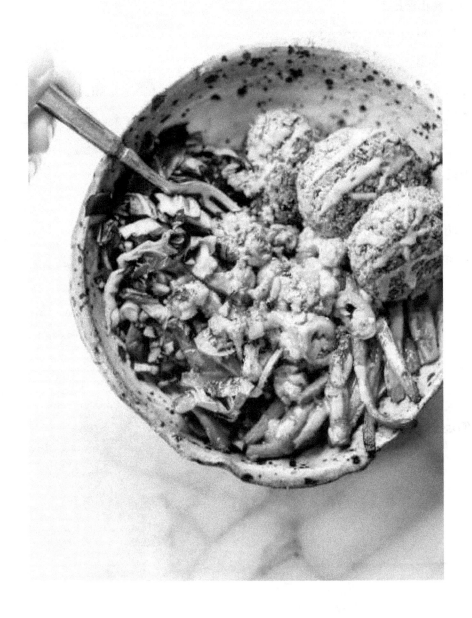

Kale Spinach and Cucumber Salad

Ingredients:

1 bunch of kale, rinsed and drained

1 bunch of spinach, rinsed and drained

1/4 white onion, peeled, halved lengthwise, and thinly sliced

1 large cucumber, halved lengthwise and thinly sliced

Dressing

¼ cup extra-virgin olive oil

2 tbsp. apple cider vinegar

Coarse salt and black pepper

Prep

Combine all of the dressing ingredients.

Toss with the rest of the ingredients and combine well.

Kale Tomato and Zucchini Salad

Ingredients:

1 bunch of kale, rinsed and drained

5 medium plum tomatoes, halved lengthwise, seeded, and thinly sliced

1/4 white onion, peeled, halved lengthwise, and thinly sliced

1 large Zucchini halved lengthwise ,thinly sliced and blanched

Dressing

¼ cup extra-virgin olive oil

2 splashes white wine vinegar

Coarse salt and black pepper

Prep

Combine all of the dressing ingredients.

Toss with the rest of the ingredients and combine well.

Spinach Plum Tomato and Cucumber Salad

Ingredients:

1 bunch of spinach, rinsed and drained

5 medium plum tomatoes, halved lengthwise, seeded, and thinly sliced

1/4 white onion, peeled, halved lengthwise, and thinly sliced

1 large cucumber, halved lengthwise and thinly sliced

Dressing

¼ cup extra-virgin olive oil

2 tbsp. apple cider vinegar

Coarse salt and black pepper

Prep

Combine all of the dressing ingredients.

Toss with the rest of the ingredients and combine well.

Watercress Tomatillo and Cucumber Salad

Ingredients:

1 bunch of watercress, rinsed and drained

10 Tomatillos, halved lengthwise, seeded, and thinly sliced

1/4 white onion, peeled, halved lengthwise, and thinly sliced

1 large cucumber, halved lengthwise and thinly sliced

Dressing

¼ cup extra-virgin olive oil

2 splashes white wine vinegar

Coarse salt and black pepper

Prep

Combine all of the dressing ingredients.

Toss with the rest of the ingredients and combine well.

Mangoes Heirloom Tomatoes and Cucumber Salad

Ingredients:

1 cup of cubed mangoes

3 Heirloom tomatoes, halved lengthwise, seeded, and thinly sliced

1/4 white onion, peeled, halved lengthwise, and thinly sliced

1 large cucumber, halved lengthwise and thinly sliced

Dressing

¼ cup extra-virgin olive oil

2 splashes white wine vinegar

Coarse salt and black pepper

Prep

Combine all of the dressing ingredients.

Toss with the rest of the ingredients and combine well.

Peaches and Tomato Salad

Ingredients:

1 cup of cubed peaches

5 medium tomatoes, halved lengthwise, seeded, and thinly sliced

1/4 white onion, peeled, halved lengthwise, and thinly sliced

1 large cucumber, halved lengthwise and thinly sliced

Dressing

¼ cup extra-virgin olive oil

2 tbsp. apple cider vinegar

Coarse salt and black pepper

Prep

Combine all of the dressing ingredients.

Toss with the rest of the ingredients and combine well.

Black Grapes and Plum Tomato Salad

Ingredients:

12 pcs. black grapes

5 medium plum tomatoes, halved lengthwise, seeded, and thinly sliced

1/4 white onion, peeled, halved lengthwise, and thinly sliced

1 large cucumber, halved lengthwise and thinly sliced

Dressing

¼ cup extra-virgin olive oil

2 splashes white wine vinegar

Coarse salt and black pepper

Prep

Combine all of the dressing ingredients.

Toss with the rest of the ingredients and combine well.

Red Grapes and Zucchini Salad

Ingredients:

10 pcs. red grapes

5 medium plum tomatoes, halved lengthwise, seeded, and thinly sliced

1/4 white onion, peeled, halved lengthwise, and thinly sliced

1 large Zucchini halved lengthwise ,thinly sliced and blanched

Dressing

¼ cup extra-virgin olive oil

2 splashes white wine vinegar

Coarse salt and black pepper

Prep

Combine all of the dressing ingredients.

Toss with the rest of the ingredients and combine well.

Red Cabbage and Tomatillo Salad

Ingredients:

1/2 medium red cabbage, sliced thinly

10 Tomatillos, halved lengthwise, seeded, and thinly sliced

1/4 white onion, peeled, halved lengthwise, and thinly sliced

1 large cucumber, halved lengthwise and thinly sliced

Dressing

¼ cup extra-virgin olive oil

2 splashes white wine vinegar

Coarse salt and black pepper

Prep

Combine all of the dressing ingredients.

Toss with the rest of the ingredients and combine well.

Napa Cabbage Enoki Mushroom and Cucumber Salad

Ingredients:

1/2 medium Napa cabbage, sliced thinly

15 Enoki Mushrooms, thinly sliced

1/4 white onion, peeled, halved lengthwise, and thinly sliced

1 large cucumber, halved lengthwise and thinly sliced

Dressing

¼ cup extra-virgin olive oil

2 tbsp. apple cider vinegar

Coarse salt and black pepper

Prep

Combine all of the dressing ingredients.

Toss with the rest of the ingredients and combine well.

Pineapple Tomato and Cucumber Salad

Ingredients:

1 cup canned pineapple bits

5 medium plum tomatoes, halved lengthwise, seeded, and thinly sliced

1/4 white onion, peeled, halved lengthwise, and thinly sliced

1 large cucumber, halved lengthwise and thinly sliced

Dressing

¼ cup extra-virgin olive oil

2 splashes white wine vinegar

Coarse salt and black pepper

Prep

Combine all of the dressing ingredients.

Toss with the rest of the ingredients and combine well.

Apples Plum Tomatoes and Cucumber Salad

Ingredients:

1 cup Fuji apples cubed

5 medium plum tomatoes, halved lengthwise, seeded, and thinly sliced

1/4 white onion, peeled, halved lengthwise, and thinly sliced

1 large cucumber, halved lengthwise and thinly sliced

Dressing

¼ cup extra-virgin olive oil

2 splashes white wine vinegar

Coarse salt and black pepper

Prep

Combine all of the dressing ingredients.

Toss with the rest of the ingredients and combine well.

Cherries Tomatoes and Onion Salad

Ingredients:

1/4 cup cherries

3 Heirloom tomatoes, halved lengthwise, seeded, and thinly sliced

1/4 white onion, peeled, halved lengthwise, and thinly sliced

1 large Zucchini halved lengthwise ,thinly sliced and blanched

Dressing

¼ cup extra-virgin olive oil

2 splashes white wine vinegar

Coarse salt and black pepper

Prep

Combine all of the dressing ingredients.

Toss with the rest of the ingredients and combine well.

Pickle and Tomato Salad

Ingredients:

1/2 cup pickles

5 medium tomatoes, halved lengthwise, seeded, and thinly sliced

1/4 white onion, peeled, halved lengthwise, and thinly sliced

1 large cucumber, halved lengthwise and thinly sliced

Dressing

¼ cup extra-virgin olive oil

2 splashes white wine vinegar

Coarse salt and black pepper

Prep

Combine all of the dressing ingredients.

Toss with the rest of the ingredients and combine well.

Tomatillo and Corn Salad

Ingredients:

10 Tomatillos, halved lengthwise, seeded, and thinly sliced

1/2 cup canned corn

1 large cucumber, halved lengthwise and thinly sliced

Dressing

¼ cup extra-virgin olive oil

2 tbsp. apple cider vinegar

Coarse salt and black pepper

Prep

Combine all of the dressing ingredients.

Toss with the rest of the ingredients and combine well.

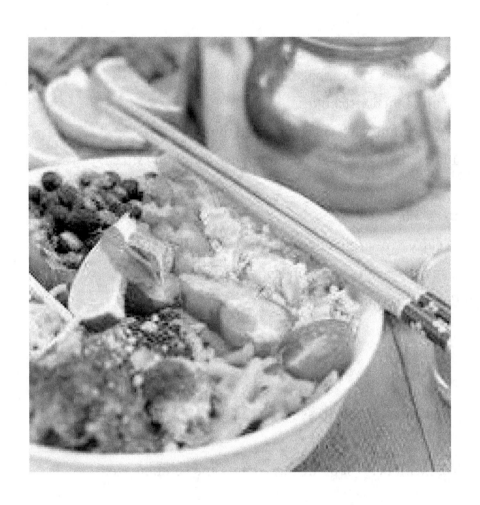

Red Cabbage Artichokes and Cucumber Salad

Ingredients:

1/2 medium red cabbage, sliced thinly

1 cup canned artichokes

1/2 medium Napa cabbage, sliced thinly

1 large cucumber, halved lengthwise and thinly sliced

Dressing

¼ cup extra-virgin olive oil

2 splashes white wine vinegar

Coarse salt and black pepper

Prep

Combine all of the dressing ingredients.

Toss with the rest of the ingredients and combine well.

Corn Red Cabbage and Artichoke Salad

Ingredients:

1/2 cup canned corn

1/2 medium red cabbage, sliced thinly

1 cup canned artichokes

1 large cucumber, halved lengthwise and thinly sliced

Dressing

¼ cup extra-virgin olive oil

2 splashes white wine vinegar

Coarse salt and black pepper

Prep

Combine all of the dressing ingredients.

Toss with the rest of the ingredients and combine well.

Ingredients:

1/2 cup pickles

10 pcs. red grapes

1/2 cup canned corn

Dressing

¼ cup extra-virgin olive oil

2 splashes white wine vinegar

Coarse salt and black pepper

Prep

Combine all of the dressing ingredients.

Toss with the rest of the ingredients and combine well.

Peaches Cherries and Black Grape Salad

Ingredients:

1 cup of cubed peaches

1/4 cup cherries

12 pcs. black grapes

1/4 white onion, peeled, halved lengthwise, and thinly sliced

1 large cucumber, halved lengthwise and thinly sliced

Dressing

¼ cup extra-virgin olive oil

2 tbsp. apple cider vinegar

Coarse salt and black pepper

Prep

Combine all of the dressing ingredients.

Toss with the rest of the ingredients and combine well.

Pineapple Mangoes and Apple Salad

Ingredients:

1 cup canned pineapple bits

1 cup of cubed mangoes

1 cup Fuji apples cubed

1 large Zucchini halved lengthwise ,thinly sliced and blanched

Dressing

¼ cup extra-virgin olive oil

2 splashes white wine vinegar

Coarse salt and black pepper

Prep

Combine all of the dressing ingredients.

Toss with the rest of the ingredients and combine well.

Kale Spinach and Watercress Salad

Ingredients:

1 bunch of kale, rinsed and drained

1 bunch of spinach, rinsed and drained

1 bunch of watercress, rinsed and drained

Dressing

¼ cup extra-virgin olive oil

2 splashes white wine vinegar

Coarse salt and black pepper

Prep

Combine all of the dressing ingredients.

Toss with the rest of the ingredients and combine well.

Watercress Pineapple and Mangoes Salad

Ingredients:

1 bunch of watercress, rinsed and drained

1 cup canned pineapple bits

1 cup of cubed mangoes

Dressing

¼ cup extra-virgin olive oil

2 tbsp. apple cider vinegar

Coarse salt and black pepper

Prep

Combine all of the dressing ingredients.

Toss with the rest of the ingredients and combine well.

Tomatoes Apples and Peaches Salad

Ingredients:

5 medium tomatoes, halved lengthwise, seeded, and thinly sliced

1 cup Fuji apples cubed

1 cup of cubed peaches

1/4 cup cherries

Dressing

¼ cup extra-virgin olive oil

2 splashes white wine vinegar

Coarse salt and black pepper

Prep

Combine all of the dressing ingredients.

Toss with the rest of the ingredients and combine well.

Enoki Mushroom Corn and Red Cabbage Salad

Ingredients:

15 Enoki Mushrooms, thinly sliced

1/2 cup canned corn

1/2 medium red cabbage, sliced thinly

1 cup canned artichokes

Dressing

¼ cup extra-virgin olive oil

2 splashes white wine vinegar

Coarse salt and black pepper

Prep

Combine all of the dressing ingredients.

Toss with the rest of the ingredients and combine well.

Tomatillos and Apple Salad

Ingredients:

10 Tomatillos, halved lengthwise, seeded, and thinly sliced

1 cup Fuji apples cubed

1 cup of cubed peaches

Dressing

¼ cup extra-virgin olive oil

2 tbsp. apple cider vinegar

Coarse salt and black pepper

Prep

Combine all of the dressing ingredients.

Toss with the rest of the ingredients and combine well.

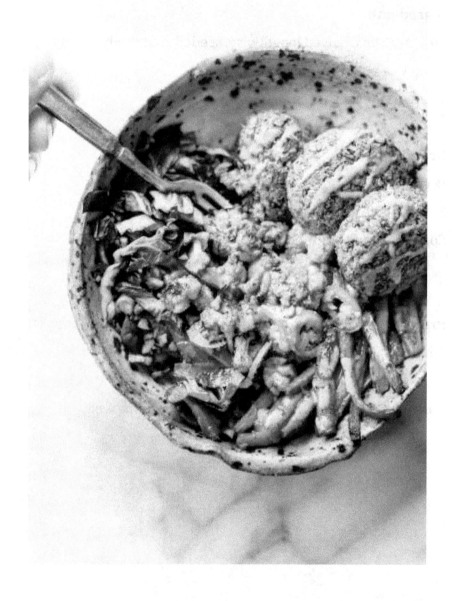

Tomatoes Pickles and Grape Salad

Ingredients:

3 Heirloom tomatoes, halved lengthwise, seeded, and thinly sliced

1/2 cup pickles

10 pcs. red grapes

1/2 cup canned corn

Dressing

¼ cup extra-virgin olive oil

2 splashes white wine vinegar

Coarse salt and black pepper

Prep

Combine all of the dressing ingredients.

Toss with the rest of the ingredients and combine well.

Red Cabbage Artichoke and Cucumber Salad

Ingredients:

1/2 medium red cabbage, sliced thinly

1 cup canned artichokes

1 large cucumber, halved lengthwise and thinly sliced

Dressing

¼ cup extra-virgin olive oil

2 splashes white wine vinegar

Coarse salt and black pepper

Prep

Combine all of the dressing ingredients.

Toss with the rest of the ingredients and combine well.

Pineapple Mango Apple and Cucumber Salad

Ingredients:

1 cup canned pineapple bits

1 cup of cubed mangoes

1 cup Fuji apples cube

1 large cucumber, halved lengthwise and thinly sliced

Dressing

¼ cup extra-virgin olive oil

2 splashes white wine vinegar

Coarse salt and black pepper

Prep

Combine all of the dressing ingredients.

Toss with the rest of the ingredients and combine well.

Artichoke Napa Cabbage and Cucumber Salad

Ingredients:

1 cup canned artichokes

1/2 medium Napa cabbage, sliced thinly

1 large cucumber, halved lengthwise and thinly sliced

Dressing

¼ cup extra-virgin olive oil

2 splashes white wine vinegar

Coarse salt and black pepper

Prep

Combine all of the dressing ingredients.

Toss with the rest of the ingredients and combine well.

Tomatoes Cabbage and Carrot Salad

Ingredients:

3 Heirloom tomatoes, halved lengthwise, seeded, and thinly sliced

1/2 medium Napa cabbage, sliced thinly

5 baby carrots

Dressing

¼ cup extra-virgin olive oil

2 splashes white wine vinegar

Coarse salt and black pepper

Prep

Combine all of the dressing ingredients.

Toss with the rest of the ingredients and combine well.

Napa Cabbage Carrots and Cucumber Salad

Ingredients:

1/2 medium Napa cabbage, sliced thinly

5 baby carrots

1 large cucumber, halved lengthwise and thinly sliced

Dressing

¼ cup extra-virgin olive oil

2 tbsp. apple cider vinegar

Coarse salt and black pepper

Prep

Combine all of the dressing ingredients.

Toss with the rest of the ingredients and combine well.

Fettuccini and Green Olives

INGREDIENTS

1 red onion, medium chopped

1 green bell pepper chopped

15 ounce can fava beans, rinsed and drained

15 ounce can navy beans, rinsed and drained

28 ounce crushed tomatoes

1/4 cup green olives

2 tbsp. capers

½ teaspoon salt

1/8 teaspoon black pepper

2 cups vegetable stock

8 ounces fettuccini uncooked

1 ½ cups Vegan Cheese (Tofu Based)

Garnishing ingredients:

chopped green onions for serving

Put all of the ingredients except for pasta, vegan cheese, and garnishing ingredients in your slow cooker.

Combine and cover.

Cook on high heat for 4 hours or low heat for 7 hours.

Add the pasta and cooking on high heat for 18 minutes, or until pasta becomes al dente

Add 1 cup of cheese and stir.

Sprinkle with the remaining vegan cheese and garnishing ingredients

Spaghetti with Butterbeans and Black Beans

INGREDIENTS

1 yellow onion, medium chopped

1 red bell pepper, chopped

15 ounce can butterbeans, rinsed and drained

15 ounce can black beans , rinsed and drained

28 ounce crushed tomatoes

4 tbsp. vegan cream cheese

1 tsp. herbs de Provence

½ teaspoon salt

1/8 teaspoon black pepper

2 cups vegetable stock

8 ounces spaghetti uncooked

1 ½ cups Vegan Cheese (Tofu Based)

Garnishing ingredients:

chopped green onions for serving

Put all of the ingredients except for pasta, vegan cheese, and garnishing ingredients in your slow cooker.

Combine and cover.

Cook on high heat for 4 hours or low heat for 7 hours.

Add the pasta and cooking on high heat for 18 minutes, or until pasta becomes al dente

Add 1 cup of cheese and stir.

Sprinkle with the remaining vegan cheese and garnishing ingredients

Spaghetti with Chorizo and Kidney Beans

INGREDIENTS

1 red onion, medium chopped

1 green bell pepper chopped

15 ounce can kidney beans

15 ounce can great northern beans

28 ounce crushed tomatoes

1/4 cup vegan chorizos, coarsely chopped

1 tsp. dried thyme

½ teaspoon salt

1/8 teaspoon black pepper

2 cups vegetable stock

8 ounces spaghetti noodles uncooked

1 ½ cups Vegan Cheese (Tofu Based)

Garnishing ingredients:

chopped green onions for serving

Put all of the ingredients except for pasta, vegan cheese, and garnishing ingredients in your slow cooker.

Combine and cover.

Cook on high heat for 4 hours or low heat for 7 hours.

Add the pasta and cooking on high heat for 18 minutes, or until pasta becomes al dente

Add 1 cup of cheese and stir.

Sprinkle with the remaining vegan cheese and garnishing ingredients

Pappardelle Pasta with Tomatoes and Vegan Cheese

INGREDIENTS

1 red onion, medium chopped

1 green bell pepper chopped

15 ounce can butterbeans, rinsed and drained

15 ounce can black beans , rinsed and drained

28 ounce crushed tomatoes

2 tbsp. tomato paste

1 tsp. basil

1 tsp. Italian seasoning

½ teaspoon salt

1/8 teaspoon black pepper

2 cups vegetable stock

8 ounces pappardelle pasta uncooked

1 ½ cups Vegan Cheese (Tofu Based)

Garnishing ingredients:

chopped green onions for serving

Put all of the ingredients except for pasta, vegan cheese, and garnishing ingredients in your slow cooker.

Combine and cover.

Cook on high heat for 4 hours or low heat for 7 hours.

Add the pasta and cooking on high heat for 18 minutes, or until pasta becomes al dente

Add 1 cup of cheese and stir.

Sprinkle with the remaining vegan cheese and garnishing ingredients

Macaroni and Garbanzo Beans

INGREDIENTS

15 ounce can pinto beans rinsed and drained

15 ounce can garbanzo beans rinsed and drained

28 ounce crushed tomatoes

4 tbsp. pesto

1 tsp. Italian seasoning

½ teaspoon salt

1/8 teaspoon black pepper

2 cups vegetable stock

8 ounces whole wheat elbow macaroni pasta uncooked

1 ½ cups Vegan Cheese (Tofu Based)

Garnishing ingredients:

chopped green onions for serving

Put all of the ingredients except for pasta, vegan cheese, and garnishing ingredients in your slow cooker.

Combine and cover.

Cook on high heat for 4 hours or low heat for 7 hours.

Add the pasta and cooking on high heat for 18 minutes, or until pasta becomes al dente

Add 1 cup of cheese and stir.

Sprinkle with the remaining vegan cheese and garnishing ingredients

Farfalle Pasta in Spicy Chimichurri Sauce

INGREDIENTS

5 jalapeno peppers

1 yellow onion, chopped

15 ounce can butterbeans, rinsed and drained

15 ounce can black beans , rinsed and drained

4 tbsp. chimichurri sauce

1/2 tsp. cayenne pepper

½ teaspoon salt

1/8 teaspoon black pepper

2 cups vegetable stock

8 ounces farfalle pasta uncooked

1 ½ cups Vegan Cheese (Tofu Based)

Garnishing ingredients:

chopped green onions for serving

Put all of the ingredients except for pasta, vegan cheese, and garnishing ingredients in your slow cooker.

Combine and cover.

Cook on high heat for 4 hours or low heat for 7 hours.

Add the pasta and cooking on high heat for 18 minutes, or until pasta becomes al dente

Add 1 cup of cheese and stir.

Sprinkle with the remaining vegan cheese and garnishing ingredients

Elbow Macaroni with Great Northern Beans

INGREDIENTS

1 red onion, medium chopped

1 green bell pepper chopped

15 ounce can kidney beans

15 ounce can great northern beans

28 ounce crushed tomatoes

3 ounces vegan mozzarella

1 tsp. Italian seasoning

½ teaspoon salt

1/8 teaspoon black pepper

2 cups vegetable stock

8 ounces whole wheat elbow macaroni pasta uncooked

1 ½ cups Vegan Cheese (Tofu Based)

Garnishing ingredients:

chopped green onions for serving

- Put all of the ingredients except for pasta, vegan cheese, and garnishing ingredients in your slow cooker.

  Combine and cover.

  Cook on high heat for 4 hours or low heat for 7 hours.

  Add the pasta and cooking on high heat for 18 minutes, or until pasta becomes al dente

  Add 1 cup of cheese and stir.

  Sprinkle with the remaining vegan cheese and garnishing ingredients

Spaghetti with Green Olives and Bell Pepper

INGREDIENTS

1 red onion, medium chopped

1 green bell pepper chopped

15 ounce can fava beans, rinsed and drained

15 ounce can navy beans, rinsed and drained

28 ounce crushed tomatoes

1/4 cup green olives

2 tbsp. capers

½ teaspoon salt

1/8 teaspoon black pepper

2 cups vegetable stock

8 ounces spaghetti noodles uncooked

1 ½ cups Vegan Cheese (Tofu Based)

Garnishing ingredients:

chopped green onions for serving

Put all of the ingredients except for pasta, vegan cheese, and garnishing ingredients in your slow cooker.

Combine and cover.

Cook on high heat for 4 hours or low heat for 7 hours.

Add the pasta and cooking on high heat for 18 minutes, or until pasta becomes al dente

Add 1 cup of cheese and stir.

Sprinkle with the remaining vegan cheese and garnishing ingredients

Whole Wheat Macaroni With Vegan Cream Cheese

INGREDIENTS

1 red onion, medium chopped

1 green bell pepper chopped

15 ounce can butterbeans, rinsed and drained

15 ounce can black beans , rinsed and drained

28 ounce crushed tomatoes

4 tbsp. vegan cream cheese

1 tsp. herbs de Provence

½ teaspoon salt

1/8 teaspoon black pepper

2 cups vegetable stock

8 ounces whole wheat elbow macaroni pasta uncooked

1 ½ cups Vegan Cheese (Tofu Based)

Garnishing ingredients:

chopped green onions for serving

Put all of the ingredients except for pasta, vegan cheese, and garnishing ingredients in your slow cooker.

Combine and cover.

Cook on high heat for 4 hours or low heat for 7 hours.

Add the pasta and cooking on high heat for 18 minutes, or until pasta becomes al dente

Add 1 cup of cheese and stir.

Sprinkle with the remaining vegan cheese and garnishing ingredients

Penne Pasta with Chorizo

INGREDIENTS

1 yellow onion, medium chopped

1 red bell pepper, chopped

15 ounce can kidney beans

15 ounce can great northern beans

28 ounce crushed tomatoes

1/4 cup vegan chorizos, coarsely chopped

1 tsp. dried thyme

½ teaspoon salt

1/8 teaspoon black pepper

2 cups vegetable stock

8 ounces penne pasta uncooked

1 ½ cups Vegan Cheese (Tofu Based)

Garnishing ingredients:

chopped green onions for serving

Put all of the ingredients except for pasta, vegan cheese, and garnishing ingredients in your slow cooker.

Combine and cover.

Cook on high heat for 4 hours or low heat for 7 hours.

Add the pasta and cooking on high heat for 18 minutes, or until pasta becomes al dente

Add 1 cup of cheese and stir.

Sprinkle with the remaining vegan cheese and garnishing ingredients

Papardelle Pasta with Fava Beans

INGREDIENTS

1 red onion, medium chopped

1 green bell pepper chopped

15 ounce can fava beans, rinsed and drained

15 ounce can navy beans, rinsed and drained

28 ounce crushed tomatoes

4 tbsp. pesto

1 tsp. Italian seasoning

½ teaspoon salt

1/8 teaspoon black pepper

2 cups vegetable stock

8 ounces pappardelle pasta uncooked

1 ½ cups Vegan Cheese (Tofu Based)

Garnishing ingredients:

chopped green onions for serving

Put all of the ingredients except for pasta, vegan cheese, and garnishing ingredients in your slow cooker.

Combine and cover.

Cook on high heat for 4 hours or low heat for 7 hours.

Add the pasta and cooking on high heat for 18 minutes, or until pasta becomes al dente

Add 1 cup of cheese and stir.

Sprinkle with the remaining vegan cheese and garnishing ingredients

Slow Cooked Fettuccini with Butterbeans

INGREDIENTS

1 red onion, medium chopped

1 green bell pepper chopped

15 ounce can butterbeans, rinsed and drained

15 ounce can black beans , rinsed and drained

28 ounce crushed tomatoes

2 tbsp. tomato paste

1 tsp. basil

1 tsp. Italian seasoning

½ teaspoon salt

1/8 teaspoon black pepper

2 cups vegetable stock

8 ounces fettuccini uncooked

1 ½ cups Vegan Cheese (Tofu Based)

Garnishing ingredients:

chopped green onions for serving

Put all of the ingredients except for pasta, vegan cheese, and garnishing ingredients in your slow cooker.

Combine and cover.

Cook on high heat for 4 hours or low heat for 7 hours.

Add the pasta and cooking on high heat for 18 minutes, or until pasta becomes al dente

Add 1 cup of cheese and stir.

Sprinkle with the remaining vegan cheese and garnishing ingredients

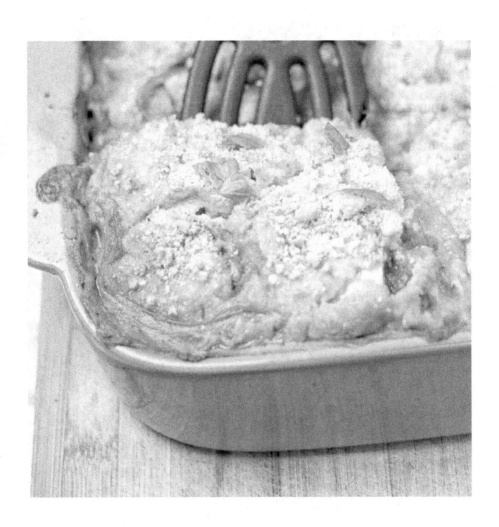

Slow Cooked Pasta Shells with Chimichurri Sauce

INGREDIENTS

5 jalapeno peppers

15 ounce can kidney beans, rinsed and drained

15 ounce can great northern beans, rinsed and drained

4 tbsp. chimichurri sauce

1/2 tsp. cayenne pepper

½ teaspoon salt

1/8 teaspoon black pepper

2 cups vegetable stock

8 ounces pasta shells uncooked

1 ½ cups Vegan Cheese (Tofu Based)

Garnishing ingredients:

chopped green onions for serving

Put all of the ingredients except for pasta, vegan cheese, and garnishing ingredients in your slow cooker.

Combine and cover.

Cook on high heat for 4 hours or low heat for 7 hours.

Add the pasta and cooking on high heat for 18 minutes, or until pasta becomes al dente

Add 1 cup of cheese and stir.

Sprinkle with the remaining vegan cheese and garnishing ingredients

Slow Cooked Farfalle Pasta with Garbanzo Beans

INGREDIENTS

1 yellow onion, medium chopped

1 red bell pepper, chopped

15 ounce can pinto beans rinsed and drained

15 ounce can garbanzo beans rinsed and drained

28 ounce crushed tomatoes

1/4 cup green olives

2 tbsp. capers

½ teaspoon salt

1/8 teaspoon black pepper

2 cups vegetable stock

8 ounces farfalle pasta uncooked

1 ½ cups Vegan Cheese (Tofu Based)

Garnishing ingredients:

chopped green onions for serving

Put all of the ingredients except for pasta, vegan cheese, and garnishing ingredients in your slow cooker.

Combine and cover.

Cook on high heat for 4 hours or low heat for 7 hours.

Add the pasta and cooking on high heat for 18 minutes, or until pasta becomes al dente

Add 1 cup of cheese and stir.

Sprinkle with the remaining vegan cheese and garnishing ingredients

Slow Cooked Spaghetti with Beans and Bell Pepper

INGREDIENTS

1 red onion, medium chopped

1 green bell pepper chopped

15 ounce can butterbeans, rinsed and drained

15 ounce can black beans , rinsed and drained

28 ounce crushed tomatoes

3 ounces vegan mozzarella

1 tsp. Italian seasoning

½ teaspoon salt

1/8 teaspoon black pepper

2 cups vegetable stock

8 ounces spaghetti noodles uncooked

1 ½ cups Vegan Cheese (Tofu Based)

Garnishing ingredients:

chopped green onions for serving

Put all of the ingredients except for pasta, vegan cheese, and garnishing ingredients in your slow cooker.

Combine and cover.

Cook on high heat for 4 hours or low heat for 7 hours.

Add the pasta and cooking on high heat for 18 minutes, or until pasta becomes al dente

Add 1 cup of cheese and stir.

Sprinkle with the remaining vegan cheese and garnishing ingredients

Slow Cooked Spicy Macaroni and Vegan Cheese

INGREDIENTS

1 ancho chili

1 red onion

15 ounce can kidney beans, rinsed and drained

15 ounce can great northern beans, rinsed and drained

28 ounce crushed tomatoes

1 ½ tablespoons chili powder

2 teaspoons cumin

½ teaspoon salt

1/8 teaspoon black pepper

2 cups vegetable stock

8 ounces whole wheat elbow macaroni pasta uncooked

1 ½ cups Vegan Cheese (Tofu Based)

Garnishing ingredients:

chopped green onions for serving

Put all of the ingredients except for pasta, vegan cheese, and garnishing ingredients in your slow cooker.

Combine and cover.

Cook on high heat for 4 hours or low heat for 7 hours.

Add the pasta and cooking on high heat for 18 minutes, or until pasta becomes al dente

Add 1 cup of cheese and stir.

Sprinkle with the remaining vegan cheese and garnishing ingredients

Penne Pasta with Pesto

INGREDIENTS

1 red onion, medium chopped

1 green bell pepper chopped

15 ounce can fava beans, rinsed and drained

15 ounce can navy beans, rinsed and drained

28 ounce crushed tomatoes

4 tbsp. pesto

1 tsp. Italian seasoning

½ teaspoon salt

1/8 teaspoon black pepper

2 cups vegetable stock

8 ounces penne pasta uncooked

1 ½ cups Vegan Cheese (Tofu Based)

Garnishing ingredients:

chopped green onions for serving

Put all of the ingredients except for pasta, vegan cheese, and garnishing ingredients in your slow cooker.

Combine and cover.

Cook on high heat for 4 hours or low heat for 7 hours.

Add the pasta and cooking on high heat for 18 minutes, or until pasta becomes al dente

Add 1 cup of cheese and stir.

Sprinkle with the remaining vegan cheese and garnishing ingredients

Pappardelle Pasta with Black Beans and Butterbeans

INGREDIENTS

1 red onion, medium chopped

1 green bell pepper chopped

15 ounce can butterbeans, rinsed and drained

15 ounce can black beans , rinsed and drained

28 ounce crushed tomatoes

4 tbsp. vegan cream cheese

1 tsp. herbs de Provence

½ teaspoon salt

1/8 teaspoon black pepper

2 cups vegetable stock

8 ounces pappardelle pasta uncooked

1 ½ cups Vegan Cheese (Tofu Based)

Garnishing ingredients:

chopped green onions for serving

Put all of the ingredients except for pasta, vegan cheese, and garnishing ingredients in your slow cooker.

Combine and cover.

Cook on high heat for 4 hours or low heat for 7 hours.

Add the pasta and cooking on high heat for 18 minutes, or until pasta becomes al dente

Add 1 cup of cheese and stir.

Sprinkle with the remaining vegan cheese and garnishing ingredients

Macaroni and Vegan Chorizo

INGREDIENTS

1 yellow onion, medium chopped

1 red bell pepper, chopped

15 ounce can pinto beans rinsed and drained

15 ounce can garbanzo beans rinsed and drained

28 ounce crushed tomatoes

1/4 cup vegan chorizos, coarsely chopped

1 tsp. dried thyme

½ teaspoon salt

1/8 teaspoon black pepper

2 cups vegetable stock

8 ounces whole wheat elbow macaroni pasta uncooked

1 ½ cups Vegan Cheese (Tofu Based)

Garnishing ingredients:

chopped green onions for serving

Put all of the ingredients except for pasta, vegan cheese, and garnishing ingredients in your slow cooker.

Combine and cover.

Cook on high heat for 4 hours or low heat for 7 hours.

Add the pasta and cooking on high heat for 18 minutes, or until pasta becomes al dente

Add 1 cup of cheese and stir.

Sprinkle with the remaining vegan cheese and garnishing ingredients

Pasta Shells with Spicy Chimichurri Sauce

INGREDIENTS

1 red onion, medium chopped

5 jalapeno peppers

1 red onion

15 ounce can kidney beans, rinsed and drained

15 ounce can great northern beans, rinsed and drained

4 tbsp. chimichurri sauce

1/2 tsp. cayenne pepper

½ teaspoon salt

1/8 teaspoon black pepper

2 cups vegetable stock

8 ounces pasta shells uncooked

1 ½ cups Vegan Cheese (Tofu Based)

Garnishing ingredients:

chopped green onions for serving

Put all of the ingredients except for pasta, vegan cheese, and garnishing ingredients in your slow cooker.

Combine and cover.

Cook on high heat for 4 hours or low heat for 7 hours.

Add the pasta and cooking on high heat for 18 minutes, or until pasta becomes al dente

Add 1 cup of cheese and stir.

Sprinkle with the remaining vegan cheese and garnishing ingredients

Slow Cooked Farfalle with Olives

INGREDIENTS

1 red onion, medium chopped

1 green bell pepper chopped

15 ounce can fava beans, rinsed and drained

15 ounce can navy beans, rinsed and drained

28 ounce crushed tomatoes

1/4 cup green olives

2 tbsp. capers

½ teaspoon salt

1/8 teaspoon black pepper

2 cups vegetable stock

8 ounces farfalle pasta uncooked

1 ½ cups Vegan Cheese (Tofu Based)

Garnishing ingredients:

chopped green onions for serving

Put all of the ingredients except for pasta, vegan cheese, and garnishing ingredients in your slow cooker.

Combine and cover.

Cook on high heat for 4 hours or low heat for 7 hours.

Add the pasta and cooking on high heat for 18 minutes, or until pasta becomes al dente

Add 1 cup of cheese and stir.

Sprinkle with the remaining vegan cheese and garnishing ingredients

Slow Cooked Penne Pasta

INGREDIENTS

1 red onion, medium chopped

1 green bell pepper chopped

15 ounce can butterbeans, rinsed and drained

15 ounce can black beans , rinsed and drained

28 ounce crushed tomatoes

3 ounces vegan mozzarella

1 tsp. Italian seasoning

½ teaspoon salt

1/8 teaspoon black pepper

2 cups vegetable stock

8 ounces penne pasta uncooked

1 ½ cups Vegan Cheese (Tofu Based)

Garnishing ingredients:

chopped green onions for serving

Put all of the ingredients except for pasta, vegan cheese, and garnishing ingredients in your slow cooker.

Combine and cover.

Cook on high heat for 4 hours or low heat for 7 hours.

Add the pasta and cooking on high heat for 18 minutes, or until pasta becomes al dente

Add 1 cup of cheese and stir.

Sprinkle with the remaining vegan cheese and garnishing ingredients

Slow Cooked Fettuccini with Pinto Beans

INGREDIENTS

1 red onion, medium chopped

1 green bell pepper chopped

15 ounce can pinto beans rinsed and drained

15 ounce can garbanzo beans rinsed and drained

28 ounce crushed tomatoes

4 tbsp. vegan cream cheese

1 tsp. herbs de Provence

½ teaspoon salt

1/8 teaspoon black pepper

2 cups vegetable stock

8 ounces fettuccini uncooked

1 ½ cups Vegan Cheese (Tofu Based)

Garnishing ingredients:

chopped green onions for serving

Put all of the ingredients except for pasta, vegan cheese, and garnishing ingredients in your slow cooker.

Combine and cover.

Cook on high heat for 4 hours or low heat for 7 hours.

Add the pasta and cooking on high heat for 18 minutes, or until pasta becomes al dente

Add 1 cup of cheese and stir.

Sprinkle with the remaining vegan cheese and garnishing ingredients

Slow Cooked Italian Spaghetti with Beans

INGREDIENTS

1 red onion, medium chopped

1 green bell pepper chopped

15 ounce can kidney beans, rinsed and drained

15 ounce can great northern beans, rinsed and drained

28 ounce crushed tomatoes

4 tbsp. pesto

1 tsp. Italian seasoning

½ teaspoon salt

1/8 teaspoon black pepper

2 cups vegetable stock

8 ounces spaghetti noodles uncooked

1 ½ cups Vegan Cheese (Tofu Based)

Garnishing ingredients:

chopped green onions for serving

Put all of the ingredients except for pasta, vegan cheese, and garnishing ingredients in your slow cooker.

Combine and cover.

Cook on high heat for 4 hours or low heat for 7 hours.

Add the pasta and cooking on high heat for 18 minutes, or until pasta becomes al dente

Add 1 cup of cheese and stir.

Sprinkle with the remaining vegan cheese and garnishing ingredients

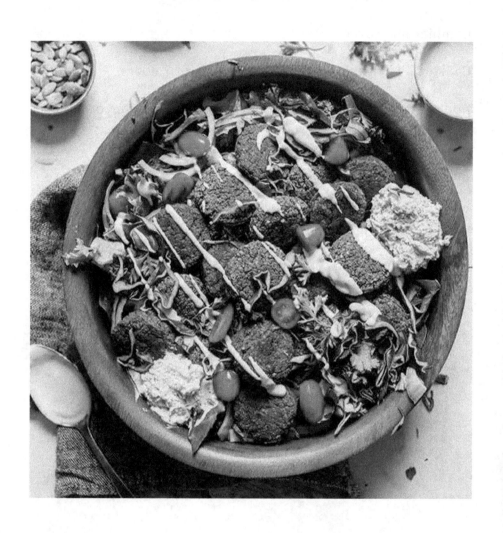

160

Slow Cooked Papardelle Pasta

INGREDIENTS

1 yellow onion, medium chopped

1 red bell pepper, chopped

15 ounce can fava beans, rinsed and drained

15 ounce can navy beans, rinsed and drained

28 ounce crushed tomatoes

2 tbsp. tomato paste

1 tsp. basil

1 tsp. Italian seasoning

½ teaspoon salt

1/8 teaspoon black pepper

2 cups vegetable stock

8 ounces pappardelle pasta uncooked

1 ½ cups Vegan Cheese (Tofu Based)

Garnishing ingredients:

chopped green onions for serving

Put all of the ingredients except for pasta, vegan cheese, and garnishing ingredients in your slow cooker.

Combine and cover.

Cook on high heat for 4 hours or low heat for 7 hours.

Add the pasta and cooking on high heat for 18 minutes, or until pasta becomes al dente

Add 1 cup of cheese and stir.

Sprinkle with the remaining vegan cheese and garnishing ingredients

Slow Cooked Elbow Macaroni and Green Bell Pepper with Vegan Chorizo and Green Olives

INGREDIENTS

1 red onion, medium chopped

1 green bell pepper chopped

½ cup green olives, drained

15 ounce can black beans , rinsed and drained

28 ounce crushed tomatoes

1/4 cup vegan chorizos, coarsely chopped

1 tsp. dried thyme

½ teaspoon salt

1/8 teaspoon black pepper

2 cups vegetable stock

8 ounces whole wheat elbow macaroni pasta uncooked

1 ½ cups Vegan Cheese (Tofu Based)

Garnishing ingredients:

chopped green onions for serving

Put all of the ingredients except for pasta, vegan cheese, and garnishing ingredients in your slow cooker.

Combine and cover.

Cook on high heat for 4 hours or low heat for 7 hours.

Add the pasta and cooking on high heat for 18 minutes, or until pasta becomes al dente

Add 1 cup of cheese and stir.

Sprinkle with the remaining vegan cheese and garnishing ingredients

Slow Cooked Pasta Shells with Capers

INGREDIENTS

1 red onion, medium chopped

1 green bell pepper chopped

15 ounce can pinto beans rinsed and drained

¼ cup capers, drained

4 tbsp. chimichurri sauce

1/2 tsp. cayenne pepper

½ teaspoon salt

1/8 teaspoon black pepper

2 cups vegetable stock

8 ounces pasta shells uncooked

1 ½ cups Vegan Cheese (Tofu Based)

Garnishing ingredients:

chopped green onions for serving

Put all of the ingredients except for pasta, vegan cheese, and garnishing ingredients in your slow cooker.

Combine and cover.

Cook on high heat for 4 hours or low heat for 7 hours.

Add the pasta and cooking on high heat for 18 minutes, or until pasta becomes al dente

Add 1 cup of cheese and stir.

Sprinkle with the remaining vegan cheese and garnishing ingredients

Slow Cooked Penne Pasta with Olives and Capers

INGREDIENTS

1 red onion, medium chopped

1 green bell pepper chopped

¼ cup olives, drained

¼ cup capers, drained

28 ounce crushed tomatoes

4 tbsp. vegan cream cheese

1 tsp. herbs de Provence

½ teaspoon salt

1/8 teaspoon black pepper

2 cups vegetable stock

8 ounces penne pasta uncooked

1 ½ cups Vegan Cheese (Tofu Based)

Garnishing ingredients:

chopped green onions for serving

Put all of the ingredients except for pasta, vegan cheese, and garnishing ingredients in your slow cooker.

Combine and cover.

Cook on high heat for 4 hours or low heat for 7 hours.

Add the pasta and cooking on high heat for 18 minutes, or until pasta becomes al dente

Add 1 cup of cheese and stir.

Sprinkle with the remaining vegan cheese and garnishing ingredients

Elbow Macaroni with Olives and Capers

INGREDIENTS

1 red onion, medium chopped

1 green bell pepper chopped

15 ounce can kidney beans, rinsed and drained

15 ounce can great northern beans, rinsed and drained

28 ounce crushed tomatoes

1/4 cup green olives

2 tbsp. capers

½ teaspoon salt

1/8 teaspoon black pepper

2 cups vegetable stock

8 ounces whole wheat elbow macaroni pasta uncooked

1 ½ cups Vegan Cheese (Tofu Based)

Garnishing ingredients:

chopped green onions for serving

Put all of the ingredients except for pasta, vegan cheese, and garnishing ingredients in your slow cooker.

Combine and cover.

Cook on high heat for 4 hours or low heat for 7 hours.

Add the pasta and cooking on high heat for 18 minutes, or until pasta becomes al dente

Add 1 cup of cheese and stir.

Sprinkle with the remaining vegan cheese and garnishing ingredients

Slow Cooked Farfalle Pasta with capers

INGREDIENTS

1 yellow onion, medium chopped

¼ cup capers, drained

28 ounce crushed tomatoes

3 ounces vegan mozzarella

1 tsp. Italian seasoning

½ teaspoon salt

1/8 teaspoon black pepper

2 cups vegetable stock

8 ounces farfalle pasta uncooked

1 ½ cups Vegan Cheese (Tofu Based)

Garnishing ingredients:

chopped green onions for serving

Put all of the ingredients except for pasta, vegan cheese, and garnishing ingredients in your slow cooker.

Combine and cover.

Cook on high heat for 4 hours or low heat for 7 hours.

Add the pasta and cooking on high heat for 18 minutes, or until pasta becomes al dente

Add 1 cup of cheese and stir.

Sprinkle with the remaining vegan cheese and garnishing ingredients

Elbow Macaroni Puttanesca

INGREDIENTS

1 red onion, medium chopped

1 green bell pepper chopped

¼ cup capers, drained

¼ cup olives, drained

15 ounce can tomato sauce

28 ounce crushed tomatoes

4 tbsp. pesto

1 tsp. Italian seasoning

½ teaspoon salt

1/8 teaspoon black pepper

2 cups vegetable stock

8 ounces whole wheat elbow macaroni pasta uncooked

1 ½ cups Vegan Cheese (Tofu Based)

Garnishing ingredients:

chopped green onions for serving

Put all of the ingredients except for pasta, vegan cheese, and garnishing ingredients in your slow cooker.

Combine and cover.

Cook on high heat for 4 hours or low heat for 7 hours.

Add the pasta and cooking on high heat for 18 minutes, or until pasta becomes al dente

Add 1 cup of cheese and stir.

Sprinkle with the remaining vegan cheese and garnishing ingredients

Spaghetti Puttanesca

INGREDIENTS

1 red onion, medium chopped

1 green bell pepper chopped

¼ cup capers, drained

¼ cup black olives, drained

15 ounce tomato sauce

28 ounce crushed tomatoes

2 tbsp. tomato paste

1 tsp. basil

1 tsp. Italian seasoning

½ teaspoon salt

1/8 teaspoon black pepper

2 cups vegetable stock

8 ounces spaghetti noodles uncooked

1 ½ cups Vegan Cheese (Tofu Based)

Garnishing ingredients:

chopped green onions for serving

Put all of the ingredients except for pasta, vegan cheese, and garnishing ingredients in your slow cooker.

Combine and cover.

Cook on high heat for 4 hours or low heat for 7 hours.

Add the pasta and cooking on high heat for 18 minutes, or until pasta becomes al dente

Add 1 cup of cheese and stir.

Sprinkle with the remaining vegan cheese and garnishing ingredients

Pappardelle Pasta Puttanesca

INGREDIENTS

1 red onion, medium chopped

15 ounce tomato sauce

¼ cup capers, drained

28 ounce crushed tomatoes

1/4 cup vegan chorizos, coarsely chopped

1 tsp. dried thyme

½ teaspoon salt

1/8 teaspoon black pepper

2 cups vegetable stock

8 ounces pappardelle pasta uncooked

1 ½ cups Vegan Cheese (Tofu Based)

Garnishing ingredients:

chopped green onions for serving

Put all of the ingredients except for pasta, vegan cheese, and garnishing ingredients in your slow cooker.

Combine and cover.

Cook on high heat for 4 hours or low heat for 7 hours.

Add the pasta and cooking on high heat for 18 minutes, or until pasta becomes al dente

Add 1 cup of cheese and stir.

Sprinkle with the remaining vegan cheese and garnishing ingredients

Penne Pasta with Green Tomatoes in Chimichurri Sauce

INGREDIENTS

1 red onion, medium chopped

1 green bell pepper chopped

1 cup green tomatoes chopped

¼ cup capers, drained

4 tbsp. chimichurri sauce

1/2 tsp. cayenne pepper

½ teaspoon salt

1/8 teaspoon black pepper

2 cups vegetable stock

8 ounces penne pasta uncooked

1 ½ cups Vegan Cheese (Tofu Based)

Garnishing ingredients:

chopped green onions for serving

Put all of the ingredients except for pasta, vegan cheese, and garnishing ingredients in your slow cooker.

Combine and cover.

Cook on high heat for 4 hours or low heat for 7 hours.

Add the pasta and cooking on high heat for 18 minutes, or until pasta becomes al dente

Add 1 cup of cheese and stir.

Sprinkle with the remaining vegan cheese and garnishing ingredients

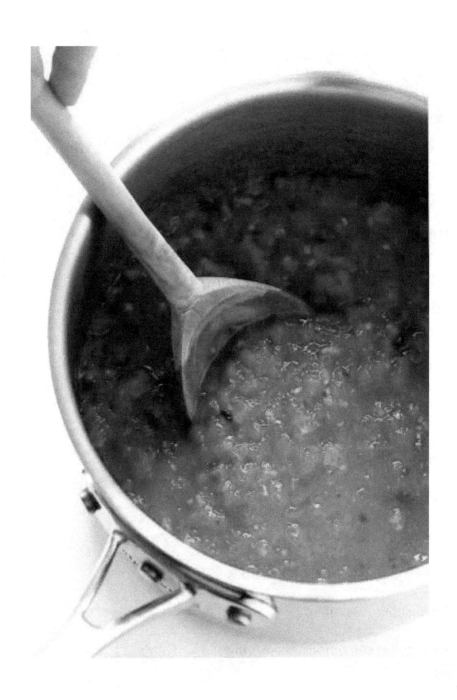

Creamy Elbow Mac and Vegan Cheese

INGREDIENTS

1 red onion, medium chopped

1 green bell pepper chopped

8 ounces vegan cream cheese

15 ounce can tomato sauce

28 ounce crushed tomatoes

4 tbsp. vegan cream cheese

1 tsp. herbs de Provence

½ teaspoon salt

1/8 teaspoon black pepper

2 cups vegetable stock

8 ounces whole wheat elbow macaroni pasta uncooked

1 ½ cups Vegan Cheese (Tofu Based)

Garnishing ingredients:

chopped green onions for serving

Put all of the ingredients except for pasta, vegan cheese, and garnishing ingredients in your slow cooker.

Combine and cover.

Cook on high heat for 4 hours or low heat for 7 hours.

Add the pasta and cooking on high heat for 18 minutes, or until pasta becomes al dente

Add 1 cup of cheese and stir.

Sprinkle with the remaining vegan cheese and garnishing ingredients

Farfalle Pasta with Vegan Cream Cheese Tomato Sauce

INGREDIENTS

1 yellow onion, medium chopped

1 red bell pepper, chopped

8 ounces, vegan cream cheese

15 ounce tomato sauce

28 ounce crushed tomatoes

1/4 cup green olives

2 tbsp. capers

½ teaspoon salt

1/8 teaspoon black pepper

2 cups vegetable stock

8 ounces farfalle pasta uncooked

1 ½ cups Vegan Cheese (Tofu Based)

Garnishing ingredients:

chopped green onions for serving

Put all of the ingredients except for pasta, vegan cheese, and garnishing ingredients in your slow cooker.

Combine and cover.

Cook on high heat for 4 hours or low heat for 7 hours.

Add the pasta and cooking on high heat for 18 minutes, or until pasta becomes al dente

Add 1 cup of cheese and stir.

Sprinkle with the remaining vegan cheese and garnishing ingredients

Pasta Shells with Tomato Sauce

INGREDIENTS

1 red onion, medium chopped

15 ounce can tomato sauce

28 ounce crushed tomatoes

3 ounces vegan mozzarella

1 tsp. Italian seasoning

½ teaspoon salt

1/8 teaspoon black pepper

2 cups vegetable stock

8 ounces pasta shells uncooked

1 ½ cups Vegan Cheese (Tofu Based)

Garnishing ingredients:

chopped green onions for serving

Put all of the ingredients except for pasta, vegan cheese, and garnishing ingredients in your slow cooker.

Combine and cover.

Cook on high heat for 4 hours or low heat for 7 hours.

Add the pasta and cooking on high heat for 18 minutes, or until pasta becomes al dente

Add 1 cup of cheese and stir.

Sprinkle with the remaining vegan cheese and garnishing ingredients

Elbow Macaroni with Red Pesto

INGREDIENTS

1 red onion, medium chopped

1 green bell pepper chopped

¼ cup red pesto

15 ounce can tomato sauce

28 ounce crushed tomatoes

2 tbsp. tomato paste

1 tsp. basil

1 tsp. Italian seasoning

½ teaspoon salt

1/8 teaspoon black pepper

2 cups vegetable stock

8 ounces whole wheat elbow macaroni pasta uncooked

1 ½ cups Vegan Cheese (Tofu Based)

Garnishing ingredients:

chopped green onions for serving

Put all of the ingredients except for pasta, vegan cheese, and garnishing ingredients in your slow cooker.

Combine and cover.

Cook on high heat for 4 hours or low heat for 7 hours.

Add the pasta and cooking on high heat for 18 minutes, or until pasta becomes al dente

Add 1 cup of cheese and stir.

Sprinkle with the remaining vegan cheese and garnishing ingredients

Pappardelle Pasta with 2 kinds of pesto

INGREDIENTS

1 red onion, medium chopped

1 green bell pepper chopped

15 ounce can kidney beans, rinsed and drained

15 ounce can great northern beans, rinsed and drained

28 ounce crushed tomatoes

4 tbsp. pesto

4 tbsp. red pesto

1 tsp. Italian seasoning

½ teaspoon salt

1/8 teaspoon black pepper

2 cups vegetable stock

8 ounces pappardelle pasta uncooked

1 ½ cups Vegan Cheese (Tofu Based)

Garnishing ingredients:

chopped green onions for serving

Put all of the ingredients except for pasta, vegan cheese, and garnishing ingredients in your slow cooker.

Combine and cover.

Cook on high heat for 4 hours or low heat for 7 hours.

Add the pasta and cooking on high heat for 18 minutes, or until pasta becomes al dente

Add 1 cup of cheese and stir.

Sprinkle with the remaining vegan cheese and garnishing ingredients

Penne Pasta with Capers and Vegan Chorizo

INGREDIENTS

1 ancho chili

1 red onion

15 ounce can tomato sauce

¼ cup capers, drained

28 ounce crushed tomatoes

1/4 cup vegan chorizos, coarsely chopped

1 tsp. dried thyme

½ teaspoon salt

1/8 teaspoon black pepper

2 cups vegetable stock

8 ounces penne pasta uncooked

1 ½ cups Vegan Cheese (Tofu Based)

Garnishing ingredients:

chopped green onions for serving

Put all of the ingredients except for pasta, vegan cheese, and garnishing ingredients in your slow cooker.

Combine and cover.

Cook on high heat for 4 hours or low heat for 7 hours.

Add the pasta and cooking on high heat for 18 minutes, or until pasta becomes al dente

Add 1 cup of cheese and stir.

Sprinkle with the remaining vegan cheese and garnishing ingredients

Garbanzo Beans with Quinoa

INGREDIENTS

6 green bell peppers

1 cup uncooked quinoa, rinsed

1 14 ounce can garbanzo beans, rinsed and drained

1 14 ounce can pinto beans

1 1/2 cups red enchilada sauce

2 tbsp. tomato paste

1 tsp. basil

1 tsp. Italian seasoning

1/2 teaspoon garlic powder

½ tsp. sea salt

1 1/2 cups shredded Vegan cheese (Daiya brand)

Toppings: cilantro, avocado.

Cut out the stems of the bell pepper.
Take out the ribs and the seeds.
Mix the quinoa, beans, enchilada sauce, spices, and 1 cup of the vegan cheese thoroughly.

Fill each pepper with the quinoa and bean mixture.

Pour half a cup water to the slow cooker.

Place the peppers in the slow cooker (partially submerged in the water).

Cover and cook on low heat for 6 hours or high heat for 3 hours.

Uncover and distribute the remaining vegan cheese over the tops of the peppers, and cover for a 4 to 5 minutes to melt the cheese.

Top with cilantro & avocado

Vegan Bolognese

Ingredients

1 large sweet red onion, diced

2 carrots, diced

3 celery stalks, diced

12 garlic cloves, minced

Sea Salt

Black pepper

1 16-ounce bag dried lentils, rinsed and picked through

2 28-ounce cans crushed tomatoes

5 cups vegetable broth

1 bay leaf

2 tablespoons dried basil

2 teaspoons dried parsley

1 teaspoon coarse sea salt

1/2 – 1 teaspoon crushed red pepper flakes

Combine the onion, carrot, celery and garlic thoroughly and season with salt and pepper.

Add in the remaining ingredients and stir thoroughly

Cook on low for 4 and a half hours, or until lentils begin to soften and sauce becomes thick.

Adjust seasoning by adding more salt & pepper to taste.

Brown Rice Vegan Burrito Bowl

Ingredients

1 red onion, diced or thinly sliced

1 green bell pepper (I used yellow), diced

1 mild red chili, finely chopped

1 ½ cups black beans, drained

1 cup uncooked brown rice

1 ½ cups chopped tomatoes

½ cup water

1 tbsp chipotle hot sauce (or other favorite hot sauce)

1 tsp smoked paprika

1/2 tsp ground cumin

Sea salt

Black pepper

Toppings fresh coriander (cilantro), chopped spring onions, sliced avocado, guacamole, etc.

Combine all the burrito bowl ingredients (not toppings) in a slow cooker.

Cook on low for 3 hours, or until the rice is cooked.

Serve hot with coriander, spring onions, avocado and guacamole.

White Bean Burrito Bowl with Chimichurri Sauce

Ingredients

1 ancho chili, diced

1 red onion, diced

1 mild red chili, finely chopped

1 1/2 cup white beans

1 cup uncooked white rice

1 1/2 cups chopped tomatoes

1/2 cup water

4 tbsp. chimichurri sauce

1/2 tsp. cayenne pepper

Sea salt

Black pepper

Toppings: fresh coriander (cilantro), chopped spring onions, sliced avocado, guacamole, etc.

Combine all the burrito bowl ingredients (not toppings) in a slow cooker.

Cook on low for 3 hours, or until the rice is cooked.

Serve hot with topping ingredients

Garbanzo Bean Burrito Bowl with Pesto

Ingredients

5 jalapeno peppers, diced

1 red onion, diced

1 mild red chili, finely chopped

1 ½ cups garbanzo beans, drained

1 cup uncooked red rice

1 ½ cups chopped tomatoes

½ cup water

4 tbsp. pesto

1 tsp. Italian seasoning

Sea salt

Black pepper

Toppings: fresh coriander (cilantro), chopped spring onions, sliced avocado, guacamole, etc.

Combine all the burrito bowl ingredients (not toppings) in a slow cooker.

Cook on low for 3 hours, or until the rice is cooked.

Serve hot with topping ingredients

Black Rice Burrito Bowl with Vegan Chorizos

Ingredients

5 Serrano peppers, diced

1 red onion, diced

1 mild red chili, finely chopped

1 1/2 cup navy beans, drained

1 cup uncooked black rice

1 1/2 cup chopped tomatoes

1/2 cup water

1/4 cup vegan chorizos, coarsely chopped

1 tsp. dried thyme

Sea salt

Black pepper

Toppings: fresh coriander (cilantro), chopped spring onions, sliced avocado, guacamole, etc.

Combine all the burrito bowl ingredients (not toppings) in a slow cooker.

Cook on low for 3 hours, or until the rice is cooked.

Serve hot with topping ingredients

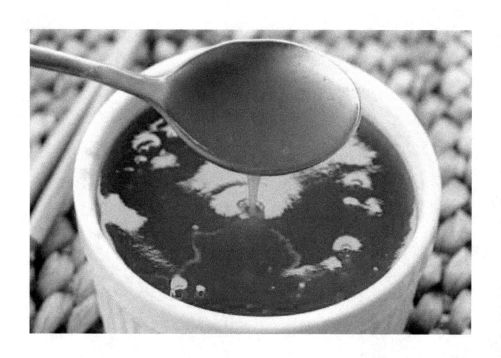

French-style Burrito Bowl

Ingredients

1 Anaheim pepper, diced

1 red onion, diced

1 mild red chili, finely chopped

1 1/2 cup white beans

1 cup uncooked white rice

1 1/2 cups chopped tomatoes

1/2 cup water

4 tbsp. vegan cream cheese, sliced thinly

1 tsp. herbs de Provence

Sea salt

Black pepper

Toppings: fresh coriander (cilantro), chopped spring onions, sliced avocado, guacamole, etc.

Combine all the burrito bowl ingredients (not toppings) in a slow cooker.

Cook on low for 3 hours, or until the rice is cooked.

Serve hot with topping ingredients

Chipotle Burrito Bowl

Ingredients

5 Serrano peppers, diced

1 red onion, diced

1 mild red chili, finely chopped

1 1/2 cup navy beans, drained

1 cup uncooked black rice

1 1/2 cup chopped tomatoes

1/2 cup water

1 tbsp chipotle hot sauce (or other favorite hot sauce)

1 tsp smoked paprika

1/2 tsp ground cumin

Sea salt

Black pepper

Toppings: fresh coriander (cilantro), chopped spring onions, sliced avocado, guacamole, etc.

Combine all the burrito bowl ingredients (not toppings) in a slow cooker.

Cook on low for 3 hours, or until the rice is cooked.

Serve hot with topping ingredients

Plum Tomato Artichoke and Napa Cabbage Salad

Ingredients:

5 medium plum tomatoes, halved lengthwise, seeded, and thinly sliced

1 cup canned artichokes

1/2 medium Napa cabbage, sliced thinly

Dressing

¼ cup extra-virgin olive oil

2 splashes white wine vinegar

Coarse salt and black pepper

Prep

Combine all of the dressing ingredients.

Toss with the rest of the ingredients and combine well.

Pickles Grape and Corn Salad

Ingredients:

1/2 cup pickles

10 pcs. red grapes

1/2 cup canned corn

1 large cucumber, halved lengthwise and thinly sliced

Dressing

¼ cup extra-virgin olive oil

2 splashes white wine vinegar

Coarse salt and black pepper

Prep

Combine all of the dressing ingredients.

Toss with the rest of the ingredients and combine well.

Tomatillos Cherries and Spinach Salad

Ingredients:

10 Tomatillos, halved lengthwise, seeded, and thinly sliced

1/4 cup cherries

1 bunch of spinach, rinsed and drained

12 pcs. black grapes

Dressing

¼ cup extra-virgin olive oil

2 tbsp. apple cider vinegar

Coarse salt and black pepper

Prep

Combine all of the dressing ingredients.

Toss with the rest of the ingredients and combine well.

Apples Red Cabbage and Cherry Salad

Ingredients:

1 cup Fuji apples cubed

1/2 medium red cabbage, sliced thinly

1/4 cup cherries

1/4 white onion, peeled, halved lengthwise, and thinly sliced

1 large cucumber, halved lengthwise and thinly sliced

Dressing

¼ cup extra-virgin olive oil

2 splashes white wine vinegar

Coarse salt and black pepper

Prep

Combine all of the dressing ingredients.

Toss with the rest of the ingredients and combine well.

Plum Tomato Apple and Red Cabbage Salad

Ingredients:

5 medium plum tomatoes, halved lengthwise, seeded, and thinly sliced

1 cup Fuji apples cubed

1/2 medium red cabbage, sliced thinly

1/4 cup cherries

Dressing

¼ cup extra-virgin olive oil

2 splashes white wine vinegar

Coarse salt and black pepper

Prep

Combine all of the dressing ingredients.

Toss with the rest of the ingredients and combine well.

Plum Tomato Kale Pineapple and Mango Salad

Ingredients:

5 medium plum tomatoes, halved lengthwise, seeded, and thinly sliced

1 bunch of kale, rinsed and drained

1 cup canned pineapple bits

1 cup of cubed mangoes

Dressing

¼ cup extra-virgin olive oil

2 splashes white wine vinegar

Coarse salt and black pepper

Prep

Combine all of the dressing ingredients.

Toss with the rest of the ingredients and combine well.

Kale Pineapple Mango and Cucumber Salad

Ingredients:

1 bunch of kale, rinsed and drained

1 cup canned pineapple bits

1 cup of cubed mangoes

1 large cucumber, halved lengthwise and thinly sliced

Dressing

¼ cup extra-virgin olive oil

2 splashes white wine vinegar

Coarse salt and black pepper

Prep

Combine all of the dressing ingredients.

Toss with the rest of the ingredients and combine well.

Tomatillo Mango and Apple Salad

Ingredients:

10 Tomatillos, halved lengthwise, seeded, and thinly sliced

1 cup of cubed mangoes

1 cup Fuji apples cubed

1/2 medium red cabbage, sliced thinly

Dressing

¼ cup extra-virgin olive oil

2 tbsp. apple cider vinegar

Coarse salt and black pepper

Prep

Combine all of the dressing ingredients.

Toss with the rest of the ingredients and combine well.

Ingredients:

1 head romaine lettuce, chopped

4 whole ripe tomatoes, cut into 6 wedges each, then each wedge
cut in half

1 whole medium cucumber, peeled, cut into fourths lengthwise,
and diced into large chunks

vegan cheese, for garnish

Dressing

1/4 cup balsamic vinegar

2 teaspoons brown sugar

1 tsp. garlic powder

1/2 teaspoon salt

1/2 teaspoon freshly ground black pepper

3/4 cup olive oil

Prep

Combine all of the dressing ingredients in a food processor.

Toss with the rest of the ingredients and combine well.

CPSIA information can be obtained
at www.ICGtesting.com
Printed in the USA
BVHW030316140722
641929BV00022B/362

9 781804 508091